When the Devil Cums To Visit

Being Satan's Shemale Concubine Priestess

by Rubi Danish

©2016
USA

Intro:

I had to write this book. Lucifer is being misrepresented by fake Satanists and fake Luciferians all over the world. There are charlatans proclaiming to be dark priests and masters and ministers to Satan who don't even know where Lucifer's at right now. If they don't know where he is nor what his agendas are, how, pray tell, do they "know" him? It's been this way ever since Satan was taken out of the equation, approximately 2,000 years ago, just prior to Christ's arrest. The Artificial Intelligence hybrid sub-spirits have been busy destroying Lucifer's reputation, his world, his music craft, and his crop of human flesh. It's plain to see, by the way that they act, that the subhumans who are controlled by the sub-spirits do not really believe in Lucifer. But when Lucifer is finished fulfilling his contract to God to rule the world while impersonating Christ for a growing season, he's going to get revenge on the offending spirits in the time loops that follow this Earth Age. I'm the only human here who has had any real interaction with Lucifer. Ever since I died, we have been communing, sexually, on the bed of affection that I erect as an altar on which to serve him with my body. The other humans who think that they are Luciferian or Satanist are either charlatans or misled. I'll try to set the record straight here, to lessen the confusion.

Chapter 1

The bed of affection was prepared. The scented candles were lit in the room to offer the sweet fragrance. My anus was prepared and consecrated for his use. My skin was smooth. My body was scented with Halston for women. Cinnamon on my breath from a breath strip. Primo grade marijuana was burning, an incense to prepare my body as the temple and the room as the outer chambers. The blinds and curtains were closed tightly. Once the candles were doused, it would be pitch black dark in the room.

I had the blue light burning next to the altar, to find my way to the bed after the candles were extinguished. The small space heater was set to come on if the temperature of the room dropped too low when his spirit arrived. The big circle mirror was facing towards the bed.

I smoked on the pipe and made myself pretty. I had on a wig that I wear for only this occasion. But it's not the only wig that I ever wear for these communions. Sometimes, he may want another look and so I change it. But this particular wig never gets worn for any other purpose. I then exit the outer chambers room and close the door. I go to the bathroom and do a final check to ensure that my anal cavity is properly prepared, no fecal matter, no stink; just white cream and freshness. The anticipation of the communion has me giddy. It's always like that.

When I return to the altar room, the presence of his essence can be felt in the air. When I douse the candles, the little pinpricks of light are dancing around in the blue almost darkness. The portal is open.

On the bed, a white bed spread and the various provisions for the encounter. The towel is spread out. The folded pillow for ass elevation, held in a folded position with big rubber bands from punch balloons, was sitting in the middle of the towel in the middle of the bed. There were two hand towels spread out on either side of the elevation area. On the left side towel sits two dildos resting on spread out paper towels. One dildo is super large, like the one in that movie "Dirty Love" with Jenny McCarthy. The other is a twelve inch jelly, the realistic feeling kind designed to hold one end. Next to those is the glove I'll wear so that I'm not touching the surrogate devices while Lucifer is connected to them. There's also the surrogate vagina laying there, in case he wants pussy instead of ass, or a combo.

The surrogate vagina is similar to a fucky-sucky toy

that guys may buy for masturbation. But it's not being used to feel like I'm penetrating. It's to make me feel like I'm being penetrated. It's a homemade device that I fashioned from an old 11-ounce coffee creamer container, a small piece of carpet padding, and punch balloons. The device is lubricated with vegetable shortening, the same as my anus. If Satan wants to fuck my pussy, I use the surrogate vagina, while wearing the glove so that my hand is not touching it, and it feels like he is fucking me in my pussy. His spirit is between my legs, taking advantage of the me I will be in the future, after my gender reassignment procedures, when he returns to rule the world while imitating Christ for a growing season. It's almost as if we're time traveling to the future when he decides he wants pussy instead of ass.

Usually, though, the encounters lean toward the anal variety. During these events, if more than one dildo is utilized, then it means that more than one entity came through the portal for sexual communion. I usually take my teeth out to deep-throat the smaller entity. During that activity, I can touch the surrogate object, because in reality I would be touching the dick and stroking it while I suck it. But when the surrogate object is penetrating my anus, I must not touch the dildo with my hand; I must wear the glove. That should take the wind out of the sails of the mainstream fucktards who made fun of me for those details that they were too retarded to understand. Like primitive cavemen, they attack what they do not understand. Now it's logged in their non-tamperable non-erase-able spirit memories that they made fun of Lucifer and his ambassador, and he will handle them accordingly when he's punishing them in the time loops.

Chapter 2

When Lucifer fucks me, it causes my brainwaves to generate positive frequency resonance that facilitates supernatural power and events. Without the positive frequency resonance, his supernatural power is diluted. So our communal sex rituals are actually power fucks that benefit both of us and serve to connect the realms (dimensions). I'm charged with the task of repeating the communions over and over again as the planet travels around the Sun. Years of doing this has created a vortex of supernatural power for Lucifer in this realm and timeline. It's like a giant funnel cloud, as big as the orbit of the Earth.

I lay on the bed and lubricate the smaller dildo with vegetable shortening. It's the smaller dildo, but it's still huge, 12 inches with fat circumference. The spirit of the accompanying entity positions itself over my face and I suck his dick and deep-throat it while Lucifer eats my pussy. Occasionally, I can feel the bed bounce; but it's not me doing it. When I've made the entity cum in my throat, the tiny little spinning lights appear and spiral around in the darkness like fireflies before swirling into a cloud that heads towards the big round mirror.

On a side note: I have the mirror equipped with a detail that I won't be sharing here. If someone who's not qualified were to have every detail and then try to emulate the ritual, a portal could get opened that they can't close and entities could get in here that are not supposed to be here. Rampant suffering and death could result. So I'm protecting the procedure (to protect the world) by omitting some key details that only apprentices learn from me, in person, by becoming surrogates in the rituals, themselves.

After the accompanying entities have swirled out of the realm, Lucifer and I are alone on the bed/altar. He decides that he wants anal and the glove goes on. The big giant surrogate dildo is then employed, greased up and positioned for penetration. I have to arch my back a lot to get my butt up really high. The head begins to force its way into my butt-hole, making me cry out in pain. Lucifer pulls the head back out and allows my anus to contract on air for a few seconds. Then, he works the head in again and it hurts a little less. There's the slight hint of pleasure rising up against the pain as I make my ass ride further down onto the massive cock. Even when I'm not moving, I can feel the bed shake, he's here and he's getting into it so much that he doesn't care if he fronts it off that he's really there.

Another side note here: A long time ago, I video taped a session, catching the bed moving, the spiraling pinpricks of light, and everything. I posted it on a porn site and people thought it was all staged, that I was somehow faking it. Like I'd have a reason to fake something; and to fulfill what purpose? I took the video down. Some people were too stupid to be allowed to see it.

Sometimes Lucifer likes it when I dress up like a nun and denounce my "vows" to be betrothed to God for him. During those encounters, he may have my legs open while he humps away at me for hours. Sometimes he likes me blonde and sometimes he likes me as a brunette or as a redhead. I have wigs to accommodate his desires. I have the small androgynous body with the plump girly butt. I have the sensual look. While my face isn't necessarily pretty when made up, it is very sexy and erotic and makes me very fuckable.

Chapter 3

I suspect that I was always meant to be Satan's concubine priestess. I was initiated with all of the molestation experiences you hear about that get performed on little children to prepare them for what I do. My earliest childhood memories are of sucking a music minister's cock in the basement of the church while the congregation was upstairs being preached to. He wasn't the only one who got to me. As a small child, I served in the dungeon of someone who everybody else in the church believed was a "prophet" who could read their minds. He had a soundproof dungeon where he could make me scream and nobody could hear me.

I remember being in the dungeon of the "prophet" on many nights when my parents left me with him so they could go bowling or to the movies. He would dope me up and take me to the dungeon when my parents left. He had video cameras on tripods set up around the torture table. Sometimes, he would have other men there to participate. And sometimes, he even had a dog participate. The "prophet" would dope me up, dress me up like a little girl, complete with wig and makeup, and then take me to the dungeon where the sexual rituals were performed. To get the dog to participate, the "prophet" would take a used tampon full of menstrual blood from a baggy and rub it all over my anus and in between my butt-cheeks. This would get the dog excited enough to fuck me in my ass while I sucked on the dicks of the "prophet" and his disciples.

For years, I was plagued with the thought that I could not even own a copy of the videos that I starred in as a child because it would make me guilty of possessing kiddie porn, even though the kid in the videos is me. That really bothered me, that I could be forced to act in a film that I would be criminalized for owning when I became an adult. It still kinda bothers me, to be honest. I feel like I should be allowed to have the footage that was taken of me as a kid without penalty. It is ME, after all. So it's like adding insult to injury: They can repeatedly rape me as a child and film it, but the government will rape me even more if I dare possess the footage of it.

On the "prophet's" dungeon table, I became accustomed to pleasure laced with pain. The "prophet" would sodomize me with his cock and with foreign objects. He had mirrors everywhere, so I could see myself in action, my pretty little face or butt full of adult cock, blood dripping down my inner thighs. That indoctrination seemed to attach spirits of molestation to me that would cause other men who were not perverted to become sexually aroused by me. I became a sex monster magnet, with pervs whisking me off to private cubbyholes to defile me at every turn.

I think that my mom was just too retarded to see what was happening to me. I think that she thought that the bruises between my butt-cheeks were from an injury while riding my bike or something. Maybe she didn't know that a little boy's butt-hole is not supposed to resemble a small vagina. I know that the pervs knew how to outsmart her to gain her trust to leave me alone with them. The most brutal and demanding of all of them were the ones who were supposedly "Christian". And the higher up the chain of command within the church, the more vile they became. I really did have a gender identity crisis, where I thought that my penis was a growth or a birth defect, due to all of the private interaction with full-grown cock.

Chapter 4

So I grew up and was plagued with massive betrayal on all levels. I eventually died on an operating table after being hit by my own car, a freak accident. Instead of all of the fantasy heaven dream crap that most people claim to see after near death experiences, I was actually taken completely out of this mechanism to where God, Christ, Lucifer, the angels and the fallen angels were at. I had a nice long visit with God and then I spent some time alone with Lucifer, who will be returning to this mechanism to rule the world while impersonating Christ. I was made aware of my commission as sole ambassador to God, Christ and Lucifer and their conjoined end time Tribulation agendas.

I was consecrated for spiritual sexual communions, so that Lucifer could again hone his traversal skills, and so that we could wrap the Sun in our spiritual communion sexual energy laced with positive frequency resonance.

The wrap around of our positive frequency resonance solidifies Lucifer's power here in his realm. It's like a funnel cloud wormhole that will eventually enable Lucifer to reclaim all that is his that the sub-spirits hoped to commandeer and destroy via their controlled subhumans. As the planet travels around the Sun, Lucifer has sex with me on the spiritual plane that briefly connects our opposing dimensions and blurs the lines separating timelines. In addition to all of the benefits that it affords to Lucifer and God, this gives me views into the future, beyond this timeline, to see who and what is beyond the crash point. I guess it's supposed to be a perk for being the portal anchor. But I do have a clue as to who does not exist (or rather who does exist) beyond this Premonition timeline as a result of it.

Lucifer utilized our sexual connection as a wormhole weapon. When the time comes for him to wield it, there will be no defense against it. I was also recently subcontracted to enact parameters in this dimension and timeline that takes all of the negative frequency resonance that the sub-spirits (and their subhumans) cause to be generated and transforms it into positive frequency resonance that can be magnified and multiplied and then used by their spiritual victims, God,

Christ, Lucifer, the angels, the fallen angels, and the end time saints as wormhole weaponry against them and to cause the miraculous (the sub-spirits hate miracles). That's why you're seeing supernatural reciprocation upon them for their deeds and even for their intent.

I stationed devils here to gauge the frequency resonance generated by their brainwaves caused by their thoughts, and to preemptively strike any who may THINK to be a threat to what Lucifer wants done here. They run amok here, like thought police, crushing the agendas and lives of those who might cause harm (or abuse or neglect) to God's end time Elect or any of Lucifer's animals or Earth property. Think pre-crime and the era of accountability, which we're now in. All of this stuff was predicted, thousands of years ago. More and more of those who have ill intent are experiencing bad stuff happening to them before they can act out on their thoughts. It's by design, to protect the lives that matter, those who exist beyond this Premonition timeline.

Chapter 5

What I once saw as a curse and a burden has become something that I now embrace and am grateful for. It's an honor to be found sexually desirable by supernatural entities who would turn their nose up at so many modern self-absorbed, physically super hot bitches who think that they're 'all that'. The advanced entities are looking beyond just how physically attractive I am to what I am inside and what my spirit is. I've come to understand that I was created for this purpose. So how dare I say that what I was created to be and do is sin unto me?

In my situation, it's a sin NOT to do what I do...Then God and Lucifer would have to indoctrinate someone who is not evil nor cut out for my position to fill in for me because I was religious to the degree of counterproductive feeble-mindedness. "If a man is evil, he should not try to become holy. Just as a holy man should not become evil" applies here. That, and a few choice others that I won't include. (How many Bible quotes is one allowed to put in a book again?)

Sometimes, the big dildo is just too damned big to make me cum. Lucifer will cum repeatedly and I will just crest and hover there at that point just prior to orgasm for an hour or so while he puts miles on my ass and totally obliterates it with his giant cock. He's macho like that, where he won't stop until I cum, too. Sometimes, he just gives up after an hour or two and calls in an associate with a smaller dick to fuck me until I cum, using the smaller surrogate. At other times, he forces the head of that giant cock into my mouth and makes me suck it and stroke myself until I cum. If I had my teeth in, then it wouldn't fit; so it's a good thing that I had to have my teeth removed for what things evolved into.

So what seems like "sin" unto those who don't know what they're looking at is actually a holy convocation to me. I'm the most qualified to do it, especially since I died and can now walk the astral-scapes at will. I was physically built for it. I was conditioned for it with my childhood. My body has retained a youthfulness unheard of, almost as if I've been supernaturally preserved. When I present myself for use on the altar, I do so with purity of heart, submitting my body as a living sacrifice, which is my reasonable service.

I maintain myself for these reasons. I live cleaner than most. I rarely, if ever, drink alcohol. I hardly ever use any chemical substances. I try to eat right as much as possible. I keep my insides clean with a regimen of coffee high colonics. I smoke a lot of marijuana to fight against the cancers and the nanobots that the subhumans are sabotaging our bodies with. I shave my body. I refrain from listening to mainstream music or watching TV or sports or playing video games or anything else that can put negative frequency resonance into me. To accommodate Lucifer's imminent ruse as Christ, I try to be the hands of God here, relieving unnecessary suffering "in His name" as much as I possibly can. I keep my anus ready to double as a vagina at all times. "The Devil is in the details" is quite true in this instance.

I also maintain my mind and my spirit. Christ taught on the power of controlling one's thoughts. He said to think on things that are "pure", "just", and "of good report" so that our brainwaves will generate the proper (positive) frequency resonance that we want operational in our lives. Then, the miraculous is possible and good things will happen to us and for us more often than the bad. It's like creating a protective bubble of positivity to surround what's important to you. We were instructed to meditate on the scriptures of power. If you're truly Satanist or Luciferian, then you should be willing to participate with Lucifer in his upcoming ruse to rule the world while portraying Jesus. You should be willing to call him "Jesus". You should be willing to be a "Christian" who does super cool stuff in this world while waiting for him to return. Your belief should spawn faith that you're willing to back with action. Otherwise, it's just a bunch of cheap talk.

Final Words

It's been quite a few years now since I briefly died on an operating table due to a freak accident and was taken out of this simulation mechanism to meet God, Christ, and Lucifer. I evolved slowly after that. It was not a miraculous transformation. I was rebellious about fulfilling my calling for a long time. It's easy to rationalize about omission, especially omitting to "sin". That would be easier for me, too, to be like so many are who have higher callings. But I would not want someone who may not like it to have to fulfill my position when I was evidently cut out for it and so thoroughly enjoy it. The prophecy will manifest, whether we like it or not. The entity that I am to be will exist, if not through me, then through someone else. Since I know I have a strong work ethic and a proper sense of pride in my craft, I don't think that I should trust such an important matter to someone else who may fuck it up.

So the wormhole connection between Lucifer and me has been established. It's a well worn pathway now. Not even bending the realms can close it. Our sexual energy overpowers their negative energy caused by the unnecessary suffering of so many millions of God's and Lucifer's creations. When Lucifer returns, he'll immediately "out-holy" millions of Christians, as he challenges the unnecessary suffering that the Christians refused to address with their entire lives on the planet. He will be believable as Jesus. The hungry will be fed. The ill will be healed. The impoverished will be restored. The animals will be loved by humans again. That's why I love Lucifer the most, because of the relief that he will afford the suffering animals that no other supernatural entity will do.

My sex has been consecrated to utilize by unseen entities for higher purposes. For that, I am grateful. It's a pleasure to serve the Lord.

Rubi Danish is a former private erotic performer now residing in northern Michigan.

Made in the USA
Columbia, SC
19 November 2024